Yoga for Runners

Beth Brombosz, PhD

This book is intended to be a general guide for runners interested in starting a yoga practice. I strongly recommend that you consult a yoga teacher if you have any questions about the poses. Your teacher will help you make sure you practice the poses safely. It's important to remember that you should never feel pain while practicing yoga, especially in the joints. Be mindful of the signals your body sends you and don't take your body doesn't to go.

CONTENTS

FOREWARD
My Yoga Story

I think a lot of people assume that yoga teachers start out practicing yoga at a very young age, living and breathing yoga with every step they take. My path to yoga was a little different. I started my yoga journey as a runner looking to get stronger and faster. I'd read all about how great yoga was for runners in several books and magazines, read that there were elite athletes who swore by yoga to help keep them healthy. After battling a mild case of Runner's Knee when I started training for my first half marathon, I hoped that yoga would help me hit a PR at my next race. I started taking classes at my school's gym twice a week and noticed that my legs, core, and upper body were feeling stronger and tired more slowly on my long runs.

It took an injury to help me realize just how much my yoga practice was helping my running. I trained for but was unable to complete the Chicago Marathon, which should have been my second marathon finish, because I injured my hip flexor. I was so busy between training, running my highest mileage yet, and writing my PhD dissertation that I gave up my yoga practice for a few months. On one of my final long runs of my taper, I started to feel pain in my hip flexor. When I had to go through physical therapy to recover from the injury, I found out that a major cause of my injury was weak muscles in my hips that weren't directly involved in running, muscles that I had been working when I was going to yoga classes.

I learned the hard way that giving up my yoga practice didn't work well for my running and my body. I began to think about how I could help other runners avoid the same pitfall. My passion for letting runners know how beneficial yoga can be for their training is what ultimately drove me to enroll in yoga teacher training. I'm now a registered yoga teacher with Yoga Alliance, teaching specialized yoga classes and workshops for athletes. I'm also a certified running coach through the Road Runners Club of America (RRCA), so I spend a lot of time thinking and writing about how runners can incorporate running into their training, knowledge that I intend to pass along to you in this book.

I realize that not everyone is lucky enough to live close to a yoga studio that offers yoga classes for runners or athletes, which is why I wanted to write this book. I hope that in the following pages I can convince you to try adding yoga to your training. And, I hope that if you do, you find that yoga benefits you as much as it's helped me.

Namaste,
Beth

CHAPTER 1
How Does Yoga Help Runners?

If you purchased this book, chances are you've heard that yoga can do wonderful things for your running. Yoga has been advertised as a great form of cross-training for runners and is a great compliment to highly stimulating activities like running. There are even elite athletes that have added yoga to their training to help them become stronger runners. I can't promise you that yoga alone will help you PR or turn you into an elite athlete, but a consistent yoga practice will help along the path to hitting your running goals. But, how exactly can yoga help you become a better runner?

Flexibility

I'll start with the most obvious benefit, the one most people associate with yoga: flexibility. If your muscles are tight, improving your flexibility can really increase your range of motion. There are some running experts who think that too much flexibility can be detrimental because holding stretches for a long period of time has the potential to reduce the power that your legs produce. Even if that's true, the other benefits of yoga vastly outweigh any potential loss in running power. Making sure that muscles aren't too tight ensures that an overly tight muscle isn't pulling on surrounding muscles, tendons, and tissues, which could lead to injury, particularly if your muscles are tighter on one side of the body than the other. Stretching sore muscles can just feel good, too.

Strength

The second benefit, strength, is so incredibly important, in my opinion. A good yoga program will work your entire body. You'll definitely improve strength in your lower body, including the muscles that you use in running. You'll also increase your upper body and core strength, which are really important to maintain proper running form, which will help you run more efficiently.

Yoga will also help strengthen the stabilizing muscles in your hips and ankles. For example, when you're holding a lunge, you're working the muscles that help to stabilize the hips. In balancing poses, you're working the tiny muscles and ligaments that help stabilize the ankle and foot of your standing leg. Yoga poses help to work stabilizer muscles for just about every joint in the body. When your stabilizing muscles are strong, you reduce the risk of getting injured when a muscle overcompensates for another weaker muscle.

Breathing

Breathing during running helps bring fresh oxygen to the cells in your muscles, allowing them to produce the energy they need to move your legs. So, it makes sense that when you can breathe deeper and more consistently, you'll be able to deliver more of the oxygen your muscles need. Any activity that can help your breathing is something that can also help your running. Yoga will help you develop those deep breathing muscles and will help you practice taking deep, full breaths to bring more air into your body.

In yoga we practice breathing, which yogis call pranayama. Working to take deep breaths helps increase our lung capacity, and we learn to keep breathing even when it's difficult, like when we're practicing twisting postures. We use our breath to carry us through tough poses, when our quads are burning or when we're working to open tight muscles. Learning to breathe through tough poses teaches you to use your breath when you hit tough, difficult patches on your runs, too.

Mental Focus

Many runners forget how much of an impact good mental focus can have on their runs, especially runs at hard effort. Learning the skills to breathe through discomfort and to push aside thoughts of doubt can help you whether you're racing or just doing a hard workout. In your yoga practice, you'll learn mental skills that will help you hold a pose even though it's tough, and you can apply those same skills to your difficult runs. When you want to come out of a pose but you stay because you know you can give a little more, you're building more than physical strength, you're building mental fortitude. Digging deep and knowing that you're stronger than you think you are will help you not only in yoga class, but will also help you at the end of a long run or in the final minutes of a race.

The Mind-Body Connection

Over time, yoga teaches you to be more in tune with your body and the signals that it sends you. With all of the distractions that most of us experience daily, it's no wonder that we tend to be pretty out of touch with our bodies. Yoga teaches us how to slow down and listen. When you quiet your mind and experience a pose, you start to come in tune with the sensations you're feeling in your body, good or bad. You'll start to notice if one side of your body is tighter than the other, or if you have a dull ache in your shin. The quieting of the mind is one of the big distinctions between yoga and stretching: you'll stretch your muscles in many, if not most, yoga poses, but connecting your body with your mind and your breath is what turns stretching into yoga.

Hopefully you're now convinced that a yoga practice can really help you improve as a runner. The next chapters will introduce you to the principles of yoga and tell you how you can begin your yoga practice. The final chapters in this book will show you yoga poses that are extremely helpful for runners and will serve as a guide as you discover which yoga poses will help you

CHAPTER 2
The Eight Limbs of Yoga

Although when we think of yoga, we most often think of the postures that we practice in a yoga class, asanas (yoga poses) are only one of the eight limbs of yoga. Yoga postures alone may give you a good stretch, but practicing the other seven limbs will help you and your running physically and mentally.

What are the Eight Limbs of Yoga?

First, a little background about where the concept of the eight limbs of yoga came from. One of the core texts of yoga is the Yoga Sutras of Patanjali. These sutras, or principles, dive into yogic philosophy in many ways, one of which is naming the eight limbs of yoga.

"Moral injunctions (yama), fixed observances (niyama), posture (asana), regulation of

breath (pranayama), internalization of the
senses towards their source (pratyahara),
concentration (dharana), meditation (dhyana)
and absorption of consciousness in the self
(samadhi) are the eight constituents of yoga."
- Sutra II.29

(Translation from BKS Iyengar's "Light on the
Yoga Sutras of Patanjali")

Let's break down the limbs a little further...

1. Yamas.

There are five yamas, or restraints, according to
Patanjali, things yogis should aspire to not do.
Those five yamas are non-violence (ahimsa),
non-lying (satya), non-stealing (asteya), non-
sensuality (brahmacharya), and non-greed
(aparigraha). Like any ancient philosophical text,
there are different ways that yogis interpret the
yamas. For example, some yogis take non-
violence so seriously that they refrain from eating

any animal products. Some remain celibate as a way of practicing non-sensuality. You get to choose how you interpret and apply the yamas to your everyday life.

There are some wonderful ways to apply the yamas to your running. For example, it's very important to practice ahimsa and to love your body as you're training. If you start to feel sick or overly sore, don't push yourself. Similarly, asteya can not only refer to stealing money or property, but also things like time. You can practice asteya when you show up on time to meet a friend for a run, or even by moving to the right side of the road to allow a faster runner to pass by so you're not "stealing" the entire path.

2. Niyamas.

The five niyamas, or observances, are things that yogis should do to in order to become good or virtuous. Those five niyamas are purity of mind, body, and the things we say (shaucha), contentment and acceptance (santosha), perseverance and austerity (tapas), introspection (svadhyaya), and study of the True Self (Ishvar-pranudhana). Again, there are slightly different ways to interpret each of the niyamas as you incorporate them into your life.

Some of the niyamas are more easily applicable to running than others. I like to think that I am practicing tapas when I push through difficult runs, finishing the workout that I set out to do. Santosha means that I accept that I've done everything that I can before a race and that I trust my training as I come to the start line. And after a race, I practice svadhyaya and think through what worked and didn't work as I prepared and as I raced, so I can learn more for the next time I train for a race.

3. Asana.

This is what we typically think of as Westerners when we think of yoga—the classic yoga poses.

Yoga asanas are meant to help the practitioner deepen his or her entire yoga practice, finding a sense of inner peace and meditation and connection with the True Self. In the sutras, Patanjali writes that practicing an asana over time allows us to calm our minds and our relax bodies in that pose as we get stronger mentally and physically. This is one of the reasons why so many yoga practitioners use the word "practice" to describe the time they spend on their yoga mat—it truly is all about practicing asanas and the other limbs of yoga.

As I mentioned before, asana is what most people think about when they think of yoga. Yoga asanas are what help you build the strength and flexibility that can help your body withstand the stress of running. Your running form improves because your stabilizing muscles are strong, helping you avoid injury. You maintain a good range of motion and help loosen tight muscles through the stretching aspects of asana. Asana helps make you a better runner physically.

4. Pranayama.

The word pranayama extends from two words:
prana, which is often described as life force, and
ayama, which means to lengthen or stretch. In
yogic traditions, breath is used to control the
prana and to help it flow properly through the
body. We become conscious of our inhales and
our exhales, how deep or long they are, the
sensation of taking each breath. However, even
if you don't explicitly believe in the existence of
prana, you can still gain a lot from pranayama
exercises.

So how can runners start to practice
pranayama? One basic exercise that I like to
lead my yoga students through is to practice
taking a three part breath. Start in a comfortable
position, whether it's seated or lying down. Place
one hand on your stomach and one hand on
your chest. As you inhale, think about pulling
your breath first all the way down to the base of
your abdomen, to the pelvic floor. Feel your belly

rise.

Once your belly is full of air, your ribcage starts to expand. Think about increasing the space between your ribs as your lungs fill with air. Your ribs expand in all directions—in front of you, in back of you, and to the sides. Finally, when your ribs are fully expanded, your chest rises. Feel your chest expanding with your other hand.

As you exhale, think about those same steps in reverse. Your chest starts to fall, then the muscles surrounding your ribs, the intercostal muscles, start to contract to pull your ribs in. Finally, your belly starts to fall as you push the final bits of breath out of your body.

Start your journey into pranayama for runners by practicing taking these deep breaths a few times a week for a few minutes at a time. Once you've mastered this breathing exercise resting, try taking these same full breaths on your runs. Practice taking deep breaths as you run. Even though you'll be breathing at a faster rate, focus on taking in more air during each breath. Through practice, you'll get better at taking deep breaths as you run.

Once you've mastered this basic type of pranayama, you can move onto more advanced exercises when you're ready, such as single nostril breathing. In basic single nostril breathing, you use your hand to close one nostril as you inhale and close the other nostril as you exhale. Surya Bhedana Pranayama, inhaling through the right nostril and exhaling through the left nostril, is heating or stimulatory. Chandra Bhedana Pranayama, inhaling through the left nostril and exhaling through the right, is said to be cooling or more relaxing. When practicing single nostril breathing, still focus on lengthening your inhales and exhales, controlling your breath.

5. Pratyahara.

Pratyahara is the practice of bringing your thoughts inward. Instead of focusing on the things you see or hear around you, you begin to instead bring your focus on your True Self. It goes beyond just closing your eyes or not touching things around you. Instead, you focus on mentally letting go of the things you sense and focus inward.

To think about how pratyahara can apply to runners, think about being at a race. There's a lot going on around you as you run—other runners, spectators, and even environmental factors like the weather. Now, imagine dropping the thoughts you have about the runner ahead of you or next to you, ignoring the people cheering for you along the course, as you begin to focus on your breathing and the sensations you feel in your body as you run. You practice pratyahara by bringing your attention inward instead of outward.

6. Dharana.

Dharana is concentration, or focus of the mind.

Dharana is what happens when we slow down and stop our thoughts and hone our consciousness on one thing, whether it's our breath or a mantra, or even a syllable like aum (om). As we practice dharana, we practice holding that focus in our minds and not letting our minds wander.

7. Dhyana.

Dhyana is most often described as meditation. With dhyana you contemplate or observe what you focused on with dharana. For example, if you're focusing on your breath during your meditation, you can consider how your lungs and chest feel as they expand and fill with air. There's also a sense of non-attachment to self with dhyana—you stop thinking about who or what you are and you just are.

Dharana and dhyana can help runners with the mental side of running, especially runners who find that they aren't as mentally tough as they'd like to be. Sometimes our minds will tell us that we can't do things that our bodies are actually physically capable of doing. When you practice listening to the signals your body sends you, you learn when your body needs a break, such as when you feel actual pain, and when you can push a little harder, such as when you're simply tired. When we're able to push a little harder, dharana and dhyana help us dig deep mentally so we can keep going. We learn to quiet those thoughts that tell us we can't run at a certain pace or we couldn't possible run another mile, harnessing the mental power we need to accomplish more than we previously thought we were able to do.

Additionally, meditation has been shown time and time again in many scientific studies to provide many benefits, including stress reduction and improved focus. If you can improve your focus and help better control your emotions while you're running, you'll be able to push through hard workouts more easily, and you'll probably be a happier person, too.

8. Samadhi.

When I was doing my teacher training, Samadhi was hard for me to understand at first. Samadhi can be described as oneness. It's cessation of thought and being completely present in the moment. Just as dhyana builds on dharana, Samadhi is the culmination of practicing dhyana. If you're mediating on an object, you mentally become one with that object. Or, if you're meditating without an object and you're mentally facing inward, you come to a place of reflection, where you're just focused on existing.

As a runner, Samadhi might be the feeling that you get when you're completely in the moment during a run, enjoying the sensation of the run and not worrying about your to-do list or even what pace you're running at. When you're able to enjoy the moment and let go of everything else, you can feel an overwhelming sense of contentment, which is what keeps a lot of runners coming back to lace up their running shoes day after day, week after week.

CHAPTER 3
Yoga and Your Training Schedule

So you're convinced that you should add yoga to your training, but what's the best way to add it in? How do you find a way for yoga to compliment your training plan but not detract from it? Following basic principles of putting together a running training plan will help you get the most out of both your runs and your yoga practice, allowing you to become a stronger runner.

But, how do you know which kinds of yoga are gentler and which are more strenuous?

Styles of Yoga

If you're interested in trying to take a yoga class at a studio, finding the right studio may feel a little daunting, especially if you don't have a studio near you that offers a yoga for runners class. Words like "hatha" and "vinyasa" can leave you feeling confused if you're new to yoga. Every studio will be a little different, but my aim here is to give you an overview of the major yoga styles that you're likely to encounter. No one style of yoga is inherently better than another, it's all about finding the right style for you.

Hatha yoga is a slower, gentler style of yoga. In a hatha yoga class, poses tend to be held a little longer than in a flow-based class, and often (but definitely not always) the poses are less strenuous than poses practiced in other styles of yoga. In many hatha yoga classes, you're encouraged to find a meditative state as you practice poses.

Iyengar yoga is similar to hatha yoga in speed in most cases. In Iygengar yoga, a strong emphasis is placed on alignment, and many Iygengar classes use many props to help maintain alignment in poses. Poses are generally held longer in Iyengar yoga than in other yoga traditions.

Flow yoga, or **vinyasa** yoga, focuses on moving between postures with your breath. In a more vigorous vinyasa class, you may hold a pose only for an inhale or exhale, but in some poses and some classes, you may hold a pose for several breaths. Vinyasa yoga includes many different subcategories of yoga, so it may be helpful to talk to a teacher or studio representative if you want to get a better idea of what a studio's classes will be like.

Technically, **Ashtanga** Yoga means any style of yoga that follows the eight limbs of yoga outlined in the Yoga Sutras. But, if you find a studio that teaches Ashtanga yoga, it almost always refers to a vigorous style of yoga that follows a set series of poses, based on the teachings of K. Pattabhi Jois. You move relatively quickly between poses, moving to your breath, as in other vinyasa yoga styles.

Power yoga is a broad term, but primarily refers to a vigorous vinyasa class. You'll move relatively quickly between poses, focusing on warming the body and preparing for more advanced poses. Some, but not all, power classes will be heated, so be sure to check with the studio you're thinking about attending if you have a sensitivity to heat.

In a **Bikram** yoga class, you practice the same 26 yoga poses in a room heated to 105°F. You'll sweat a lot in a Bikram class, so be sure to drink plenty of water before and after class. There are some studios that practice a style of yoga that's almost identical to Bikram yoga but have stepped away from the Bikram name due to the controversy surrounding Bikram Choudhury himself in recent years.

Restorative yoga, also called **yin** yoga, is a very slow form of yoga. You may hold a pose for several minutes as your muscles and connective tissue relax and release. Like Iyengar classes, many restorative yoga classes will use props to allow you to relax more into the poses since you're holding them for longer periods of time.

Taking Class at a Yoga Studio

If you're interested in taking a class at a yoga studio, don't be intimidated by visions of extremely flexible yogis. Almost every yoga studio will accommodate yogis of all levels, and many offer classes for beginners, where you may feel more comfortable. If you're nervous about taking your first studio class, these tips may help put your mind at ease.

Don't worry about everyone looking at you or not knowing every pose. I see a lot of nervous beginners come to classes looking very self-conscious. What they may not know is that no one is judging them for not being able to get into advanced poses because we were all there at some point. Yogis want everyone to feel comfortable and to come to love yoga as much as we do. We don't come to our mats to judge each other, we come to our mats to find that meditative space. Besides, the really limber yogi next to you is concentrating more on his or her own form than yours.

Check the studio's schedule for beginner's classes or workshops. Starting in a slower paced class is never a bad idea, especially if you're really new to yoga. Often classes for beginners will address more corrections to alignment which will help keep you safe on your mat and make it less likely that you'll get injured. You might also feel more comfortable at a beginners' class, allowing yourself to relax more and letting your mind go, which is the core of yoga. If you do find yourself at an all-levels class, just take it easy and modify when necessary. Many runners have the tendency to push themselves into poses that their bodies aren't ready for, which is a recipe for injury. It's better to take it easy in a pose than to take it too far.

Listen to your body! I can't stress this one enough, especially to runners who may be thinking about attending their first yoga class. Runners tend to be very tight in the hips, hamstrings, and other areas of the body and stretching too much can actually hurt you. You should never feel pain in a yoga pose. If you do, gently back out of the pose. In the style of yoga I teach, child's pose is always an option and I always encourage my students to come back to child's pose for a few breaths if they need to reconnect their minds with their breath.

Come to class early. This is true if you're just trying out a new studio for the first time, too. You'll have to sign a liability waiver and fill out some information for the studio, and you don't want to walk into class late because you were filling out paperwork. Try to plan accordingly. Arriving early will also allow you to have time to figure out where everything is in the studio (bathrooms, water fountain, if they have one, etc.)

Bring water, and possibly a towel, too. Some studios will charge you if you want a bottle of water, if you need to borrow a mat, or for other things you might need for class. Check with the studio you plan to attend to find out what their policy is and to find out what you should bring to your class, or make sure that you'll have money to get the supplies you need.

When Should Runners Practice Yoga?

Timing is incredibly important when stretching as part of a yoga practice. It's best to avoid static stretching, like what we do in yoga, before a run, but yoga is well-suited for post-run stretching. Holding stretches before a run can make your muscles contract less forcefully, so definitely don't practice yoga immediately before running a race or you may not run as quickly as you had hoped you would.

If you're practicing yoga at home after a run or on a day when you're not running, be sure that you're not practicing yoga with cold muscles. As a general rule, you want to make sure your muscles are warm before you stretch them. In a yoga class, the teacher usually incorporates warming up your muscles at the start. If you're leading yourself through poses at home, do so after a workout, like after a run or a walk. Or, you could warm your body up with some gentler yoga like modified Sun Salutations. Pay careful attention to the signals your body is sending you and make sure you're finding a comfortable stretch. You shouldn't ever feel like you're straining to hold a pose.

How Do You Add Yoga to Your Training Schedule?

Most running training plans are built upon the hard/easy rule. Your body needs to rest in order to recover from hard workouts, which is why almost every training plan you find will alternate hard efforts (speed work, long runs) with easy efforts (short, slower runs). By spacing easy workouts between hard workouts, you make sure that your body has enough time to recover and repair your muscles so you become a better and stronger runner.

Yoga should be incorporated into your training

plan just like you would add in a running workout. If you're starting your yoga journey, taking a vigorous power yoga class on an easy day would be a bad idea. Instead of giving your body the rest it needs, you would be pushing your muscles to work hard. But, a gentle restorative yoga class on an easy day could be just what your body needs. Think about whether the style of yoga is more vigorous or milder, and apply the hard/easy rule to cross training activities like yoga just like you would your runs.

Here's an example of how you might add yoga to a training program:

Training Plan Without Yoga
Monday: Rest
Tuesday: Intervals
Wednesday: Easy Run
Thursday: Tempo Run
Friday: Rest
Saturday: Easy Run
Sunday: Long Run

Training Plan With Yoga

Monday: Rest

Tuesday: Intervals + 10 minutes Hatha Yoga

Wednesday: Easy Run

Thursday: Tempo Run + 30 minutes Power Yoga

Friday: Rest

Saturday: Easy Run + 30 minutes Hatha Yoga

Sunday: Long Run + 60 minutes Restorative Yoga

The more strenuous yoga workouts are placed on the same days as the harder running workouts so the hard days incorporate the hard efforts with yoga as well. When following a plan like the plan above, always pay attention to the signals your body sends you in your yoga class. If your body feels tired from a tough workout earlier in the day, modify the asanas as needed. Pushing through a yoga class isn't worth the risk of getting injured by overexerting or overextending yourself in a yoga pose. Also, don't add in too much yoga too quickly, especially more intense forms of yoga like power yoga. Start by adding in a class or two a week and increase from there.

CHAPTER 4
Equipment

If you do a quick search about yoga equipment, you'll probably be really overwhelmed by the amount of yoga "stuff" available. What do you really need and what can you do without? Where should you splurge and where can you get away with a cheaper item?

Absolute Must: A Mat. If you have a little extra money, spend it on a good mat. Your mat is going to be your constant companion through your practice and a good mat can help you love or hate yoga. Having the right yoga mat can really change your practice. I started out with a very cheap mat that I got as part of a weight and fitness set from one of the big box stores and thought it was normal for my knees to hurt and to feel uncomfortable on my mat. When I started taking classes at my school's gym during grad school, I upgraded a bit and got an intermediate mat. It was okay, but I slipped all the time. I finally upgraded and got what I consider to be a very nice mat after a while, and this is the mat that I still use almost every time I practice. A good mat really is worth the investment. But, what exactly should you look for when you choose a yoga mat?

Quality. You really do get what you pay for with a yoga mat. I'm not saying that you have to go out and spend over $100 for a mat, but inexpensive mats are also often cheaply made. I've been to yoga studios that have very cheap yoga mats as loaner mats and people knock out small chunks of the foam the mat's made out of all the time with their rings or fingernails. It's better to spend a little more on a mat that's going to last you a while.

Materials. The most popular materials I've seen to make mats are foam and rubber. I've owned both and I've had better luck personally with the rubber-based mats. I find them to be less slippery and I think they hold up better over time. The downside to a rubber-based mat is that it can smell like rubber for a while, but I promise that smell does go away over time. If you really don't want a rubber mat (or are allergic to rubber) but slip on the foam mats, consider getting a yoga towel. If you do, I'd recommend getting one with little grips on the bottom so your towel doesn't wind up sliding all over your mat, which is very annoying (trust me).

Thickness. The thinner the mat, the less padding you'll have for your joints, especially when those joints are resting on the floor, like a lunge with your back knee on the mat. But, highly padded mats are often heavier, and it can also be tough to practice balancing poses on them because there's so much mat between you and the floor. One's not inherently better than the other; it's important to find the mat that fits your needs.

Length. If you're very tall, you might consider getting an extra long mat. Many, if not most, companies make them these days. Most standard mats are 72 inches long, give or take an inch or two, and long yoga mats often around 80 inches long. So, if you're over 6 feet tall (or 1.8 m tall for those of you not in the US), you might consider getting a longer mat.

Weight. Many of the features I've described will contribute to the weight of a mat. Foam mats are generally lighter than rubber mats. Thicker mats have more material and will generally be heavier than thinner mats. If you have a short walk from your car to your yoga studio, weight may not matter much, but if you have to carry your mat longer distances, a lighter mat may be helpful.

To summarize, to choose a yoga mat that's the right one for you, it's helpful to think about what you need from a yoga mat: more padding for the joints? Lightweight and portable? Then, choose a mat based on those needs. It's all about finding the right mat for *you.*

Might Need: A Yoga Towel. If you're not using a grippy mat, or even if you are but you're practicing yoga in a heated environment, you might want a yoga towel. Some towels have non-slip material on the bottom to help them stay stuck to your mat so they don't bunch up as you're practicing. I've personally had better luck with those towels than the towels that don't have the sticky underside. Bottom line: if you're slipping a lot, try a towel. You can rent them from some studios, or some even let you borrow one for free, which would let you see if you think one would really help you.

Must Have: Yoga Blocks (or Similar Support). I strongly recommend that runners have a set of yoga blocks as they start practicing, or at least something solid to use to help support themselves through poses like a sturdy stack of books. As a runner, I'm sure you know that running has a tendency to tighten muscles. So, if you've been running for a while, chances are your muscles are pretty tight, and your poses probably won't look like the yogi on the cover of the yoga magazine. That's perfectly fine. The important thing is that you modify the poses so that they are comfortable in your body, and one of the best ways to modify is to have something solid like a yoga block to help bring the ground up to you when necessary.

I have both cork and foam yoga blocks and my cork blocks are my favorite of the two. They were relatively inexpensive and the cork really supports you better than the foam when you're using them as props. If you plan on doing any practicing at home at all, you really should have at least one block to help you modify poses. It's better to have a block and not use it than to not have one and injure yourself because you took the pose too far.

Might need: A Strap. Yoga straps are another great way to modify poses and to help you reach into certain poses when you're not quite flexible enough to get into them yet. A belt and a hand towel can do in a pinch, depending on what length you need the strap to be. I would strongly suggest having these alternate options available if you don't want to purchase a yoga strap. Just like yoga blocks will help you achieve poses that you might be too tight to try otherwise, straps can help assist you into poses, too. Another option would be to get a yoga mat sling that doubles as a yoga strap.

Probably Won't Need Yet: A Yoga Blanket. I have a special blanket that I use for yoga and I love having it, but then again, I'm a yoga teacher. You can easily get away with using a throw blanket that you have lying around. I would strongly recommend keeping a blanket handy as you practice yoga just in case you need it for support, especially if you're practicing more restorative poses. It's a good idea to have a few pillows around for restorative yoga, too.

CHAPTER 5
Yoga Poses for the Lower Body

Most runners who want to start practicing yoga immediately start with yoga poses for the legs and hips. It makes sense—we think of our legs as the primary muscles that we use while we run. And, having good flexibility and strength in the legs and the hips is very important. Weak hips are the root of so many running injuries: as your hip stabilizing muscles get weak, other muscles take over to help control the hips when you run, leading to overuse injuries. Imbalances in the strength of muscles can also travel up and down the body, so a problem that's rooted in your hip could actually manifest itself as knee pain. Therefore it makes a lot of sense that we want to keep our legs balanced and happy by keeping the leg and hip muscles strong and by making sure we have equal flexibility on each side of our bodies.

These poses featured here aren't an exhaustive list of every yoga pose that exists, but they are poses that work incredibly well for runners and that can be modified if you have very tight muscles, something that runners often need. In any yoga pose, if a muscle is being stretched, you should feel the stretch in the middle, or the belly, of the muscle. It should feel like a nice, comfortable stretch. If you feel like you're straining to get into a pose, modify it until your body has opened enough to try the full pose. For each pose, hold for several breaths, or for as long as is comfortable.

When you're practicing these poses, be sure to remember your pranayama. One of the big differences between just stretching and practicing yoga is the use of breath as you are practicing the asanas. Be sure you are taking big long inhales and exhales as you practice each of these poses.

Leg and Hip Strengtheners

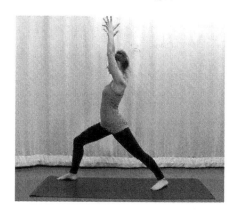

Warrior I (Virabhadrasana I) is great for building strength through the lunging leg and opening up the back side of your back leg. To find your Warrior I, begin with your legs long on your mat. The toes of your front leg point forward and the toes of your back leg point at a 45 degree angle toward the top corner of your mat. Ideally your heels should be in line with each other front to back, but if this feels unsteady, you can bring your feet closer to the long edges of your mat. Make sure your front knee doesn't come in front of your ankle. Try to bring your hips square by pulling the back hip forward. You may need to shorten your stance and bring your feet in closer lengthwise to properly square your hips.

Bringing your hips square is tough, but it can help you get a nice stretch through your calf muscles.

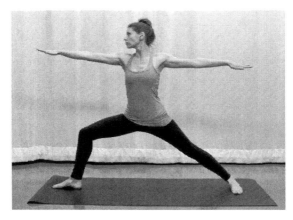

Warrior II (Virabhadrasana II) not only helps strengthen the front leg that's in the lunge, but also helps open the hips. Start with your feet long on your mat. Your front toes point to the front of the mat and your back foot is parallel to the short edge of your mat. The heel of your front foot should line up with the arch of your back foot. Lengthen your stance (bring your feet closer to the short edges of the mat) to deepen your lunge, making sure that your front knee does not come forward of your front ankle. Track your front knee toward the middle toe of your front foot. Pull your shoulder blades together and keep your shoulders melted away from your ears. Your arms are straight as you gaze over the middle finger of your front hand.

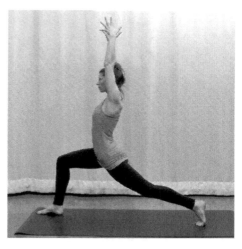

Crescent Lunge (Anjaneyasana variation) is another pose that's great for both building strength and opening the hips. With your legs long on your mat, all toes pointing toward the front of your mat. Bend your front knee so your front leg is in a lunge, knee stacking over ankle. Your back heel is lifted and your heel stacks over your toes. To challenge yourself, see if you can get your front thigh parallel to your mat while still keeping proper alignment.

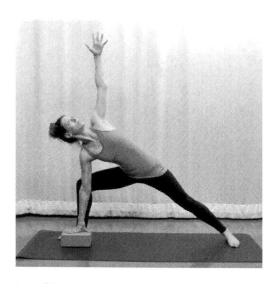

Extended Side Angle Pose (Utthita Parsvakonasana) is also great for building strength in the thigh while helping to open through the spine and shoulders. Begin in Warrior II with your right leg forward, then place your right elbow on top of your right knee, bringing your left hand up to the ceiling. If you would like to deepen the pose, you can bring your right hand down to a block or to the mat. If your hand is at a block or the mat in front of your right knee, press your right knee out with your right elbow for an extra hip opener. Think about pulling your top shoulder back to deepen the twist. Switch and hold for an equal amount of time on the left side.

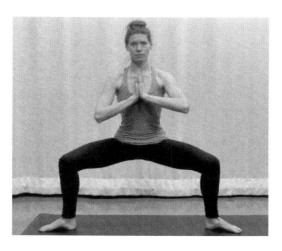

Goddess Pose (Utkata Konasana) will help you get strong through the tops of your thighs and through your hips. To begin, stand facing the long edge of your mat. Bring your legs wider than your hips, and turn your heels in slightly as your toes turn out slightly. Bend your knees and sink into a squat, keeping your knees stacked over your ankles, or slightly inside your ankles.

Work up to getting your thighs parallel to your mat over time. You can keep your hands at heart center, or you can take a 90 degree bend in your elbows for cactus or goal post arms, your upper arms parallel to your mat.

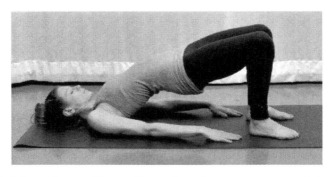

Bridge Pose (Setu Bandha Sarvangasana) is wonderful for building strength through the glutes and hips. Begin on your back with your arms long at your sides. Walk your feet into your seat so that your fingertips lightly graze the backs of your heels. Plant down firmly through your feet and lift your hips up. Try to keep your knees at hip width, or the distance where your thigh bones meet your hips, usually about two fists' distance apart.

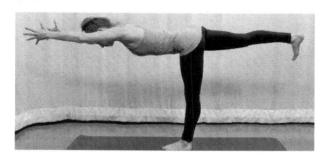

Another wonderful pose for building strength in your glutes is **Warrior III (Virabhadrasana III).** Begin in Crescent Lunge. Start to shift your weight into your front foot and leg, then lift your back leg up off the mat. Flex your back foot and straighten your back leg; feel like you're kicking something behind you. Bring your arms up straight by your ears, making a capital T with your body. Try to keep both hips pointing down toward your mat.

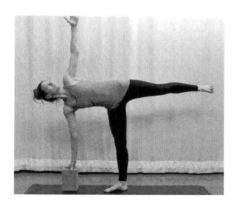

Half Moon Pose (Ardha Chandrasana) is also a balancing pose that will help you strengthen your hips and glutes. Begin in Warrior II, right foot forward. Start to shift your weight into your right foot. Lift your left leg, keeping it straight, as you bring your right hand down to a block or to your mat, depending on your flexibility. Work on bringing your hips square to the long edge of your mat, stacking your top hip over your bottom hip. Your top shoulder stacks over your bottom shoulder and bottom hand. Flexing strongly through the top leg and keeping it straight will help strengthen your glutes, especially in the top leg. Hold on the right for a few breaths, then switch to the left side.

Hip Openers

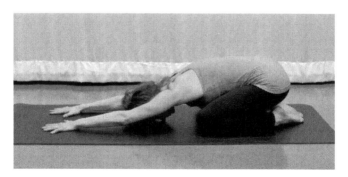

Child's Pose (Balasana) is not only a wonderful relaxation pose, but it's also a good hip opener. You will open through the hips more if you bring your knees closer to the long edges of the mat, bringing your knees wider apart. If you're very tight, bring a yoga block or another support like a folded blanket under your forehead to help support you. You can also take a blanket under your knees and/or between your seat and your thighs to help take pressure off your knees. Think about relaxing through the inner thighs, seeing if you can sink your seat closer to your heels.

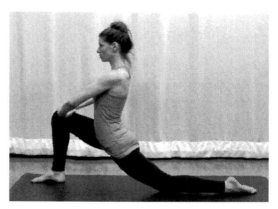

Low Lunge (Anjaneyasana) is a perfect pose to start opening the hips. Start with your feet long on your mat, both toes point forward. Shift your weight forward, bending your front knee. Bring your back knee to the mat, placing a blanket or other padding under the back knee if you need to. Your hands come to your front knee as you press your hips forward. You should feel a nice stretch through the hip flexor of the back leg. Be sure to hold the pose for an equal amount of time on the other side.

Pigeon Pose is always a favorite for runners because it helps open through the hip muscles that almost always get very tight in runners. However, because those muscles tend to be very tight, Half Pigeon Pose may be too intense. I recommend that runners start with **Reclining Pigeon Pose**, also called **Eye of the Needle Pose (Supta Kapotasana)**.

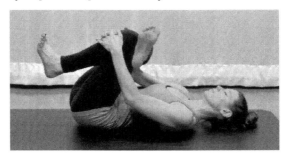

To come into Reclining Pigeon Pose, stack your right ankle on top of your left thigh, just below the knee. Flex both feet. Reach through the opening between your legs and grab your left shin or thigh. Pulling the legs into your body more tightly will intensify the pose. Be sure to hold for an equal amount of time on the other side.

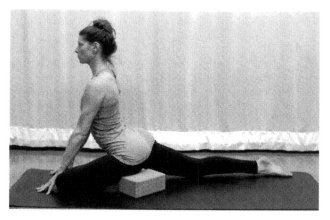

Half Pigeon Pose (Ardha Kapotasana) can provide a deeper stretch than reclining pigeon. Begin in Downward Facing Dog. Sweep your right heel up and bring your right leg forward, keeping your left leg long behind you on the mat. Work to bring your right shin parallel to the mat, although your shin will only truly be parallel if your hips are very open. You have an option to bring a block, blanket, or other support under your right hip to make the pose a little easier. Look over your right shoulder to square your hips and to make sure your left leg is straight behind you. If your hips are tight, you may have to stay with your hands on the mat or bring your forehead to a block to start. Over time, you'll loosen up and you'll be able to deepen the pose, eventually bringing your forehead to the mat. It's all about finding the right amount of stretch for where your body is that day. Be sure to practice the pose for an equal amount of time with your left leg forward.

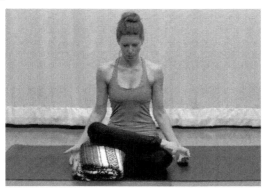

To intensify, try **Double Pigeon**, also called **Fire Log Pose** or **Square Pose (Agnistambhasana)**. This pose is very intense, but it really loosens the hips up a lot more when you've gotten the hang of half pigeon and you'd like to go a little deeper. To come into Double Pigeon, begin in a seated position. Bring your left leg parallel to the edge of your mat, 90 degree bend in your left knee with your foot flexed. Bring your right leg on top of the left, stacking your right shin over your left shin. Be sure to flex your right foot to keep your ankle straight; relaxing your ankle and letting it fall in toward the bottom knee puts too much stress on the ankle. As you work on opening your hips, it may be helpful to place a blanket or other support under your top knee to reduce the stress placed on your knees. Be sure to practice the pose with your left leg on top before finishing.

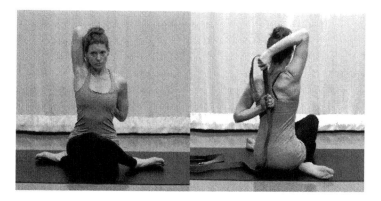

Cow Face Pose (Gomukhasana) is a great hip opener, although the full pose can be very intense if you have tight shoulders. It's fine to do the pose without the arms, or to modify. To come into Cow Face Pose on the right side, start in a seated position, then bring your left heel close to your right hip. Bring the right leg on top, bending your leg, working to get your knees to stack. If your hips are very tight, your knees may not stack—that's okay. You can play around with bringing your feet closer to your seat or to your knees to find the right intensity in the hip stretch.

To come into full Cow Face Pose, bring your right arm up above your head as your left arm comes out to your left side. Bend both elbows and bring your hands in close to each other. If your shoulders are open you may be able to bring your fingertips to touch. If not, you can use a strap or towel between your hands to help make this arm position easier. As you practice this pose, work to bring your hands closer together.

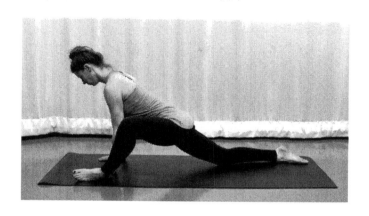

Lizard Lunge (Utthan Pristhasana) is a
wonderful hip opener, made even better by the
fact that you can make this pose more or less
active. Begin in Low Lunge, having an option to
keep your front foot where it is or slowly inch
your foot toward the top corner of your mat.
Come to the knife edge (the outside edge) of
your front foot, letting your knee fall open to the
side to stretch through the outer hip of your front
leg. You can keep your bottom knee on the mat
(or on a blanket for extra support) or you can lift
onto the toes of your back leg to work on
strength. Practice Lizard Lunge on both sides.

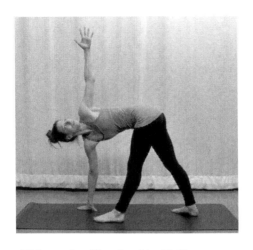

Twisting Triangle (Parivrtta Trikonasana) is a more challenging pose, but it's great for stretching out the IT band. Start by facing the front of your mat, then step your left leg back, your left foot at a 45 degree angle with your toes pointing toward the top corner of your mat. Start with just a short space between your front foot and your back foot, maybe the length of your thigh bone. Widening your stance—moving your feet toward the left and right (long) edges of your mat—can give you a more stable base for this pose. Hinge forward with a flat back, bringing your hands to a block or to the mat. Bring your left hand directly below your left shoulder, on a block or your mat, then bring your right hand high as you inhale, twisting your heart toward your right leg as you exhale. Think about lengthening your spine with each inhale and twisting a little more with each exhale if that feels good in your body. Bring your right hand back down, then switch sides.

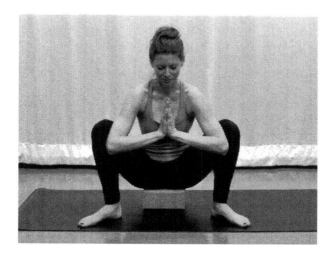

Garland Pose (Malasana) is wonderful for opening the inner thighs. Start with your feet slightly wider than your hips, toes turned out. Sink down, bringing your hips between your legs, always having an option to take a seat on a yoga block or a folded blanket for extra support. Try to keep your shoulders stacked over your hips, avoiding leaning forward too much. Bring your hands heart center and use your elbows to press your knees open for an extra stretch.

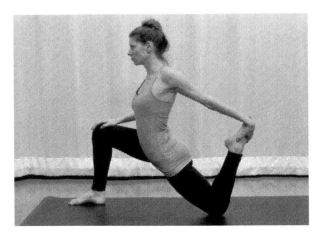

Most runners' quadriceps get tight as they run, so it's nice to have a good way to stretch the quadriceps and open the front of the leg. This lunge variation, **Low Lunge with Quadriceps Stretch (Anjaneyasana variation)**, will help you do just that. Starting in Low Lunge, simply bend the knee of your back leg to bring your foot closer to your body. If you feel a good stretch, stay there. If your quads are a little longer, you can grab your foot and pull it in, always making sure to find a comfortable stretch, never straining. You always have an option to place a blanket under your back knee for extra support and padding.

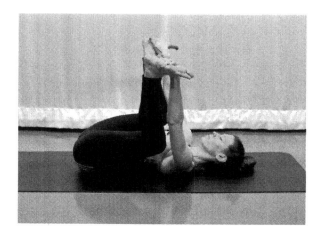

Happy Baby (Ananda Balasana) is not only a great hip opener, but it's also just plain fun to practice. Begin on your back, bringing your knees to either side of your rib cage. Bring your knees to a 90 degree bend and flex your feet. Bring your arms to the inside of your legs and wrap your hands around your feet, grabbing onto the edges of your feet. You have the option to pull with your arms to press your lower back into the mat. Once you're in the pose, you can either stay still (sometimes called **Dead Bug**), or you can slowly and gently rock side to side.

Hamstring Stretches

Many of us have very tight hamstrings. For athletes, especially runners, the hamstrings get tight as they're used during workouts. Hamstrings can also tighten up from sitting all day, which many people do in this technology-oriented world. Doing some yoga for hamstrings poses can help you loosen the hamstrings, allowing better range of motion and comfort. In all of these poses, be sure to engage your quadriceps so you don't lock and/or hyperextend your knees. For all hamstring stretches, be sure you're feeling a nice, comfortable stretch in the belly of the muscle, its widest part.

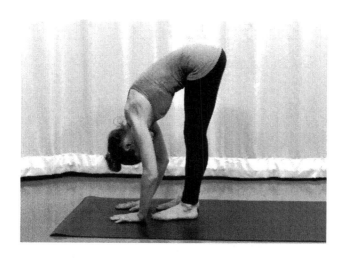

Standing Forward Fold (Uttanasana) is probably the best known yoga pose to stretch the hamstrings. You have an option to keep your feet hip width apart, or to bring your feet together so your big toes touch. In the Forward Fold you should try to keep your back straight and pull your chest toward your legs—don't curl your back over and just try to get your nose to your legs. To modify for tight hamstrings, bend your knees more and place a yoga block or other firm object beneath your hands.

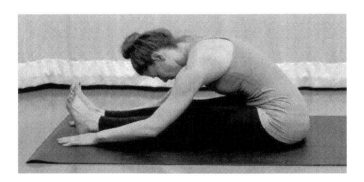

Seated Forward Fold (Paschimottanasana) is another forward fold variation that's wonderful for helping to lengthen the hamstrings. To come into Seated Forward Fold, take a seat on your mat, zip your legs together, flex your feet, then carefully fold forward. As in Standing Forward Fold, try to keep your back as flat as possible and think about pulling your chest to your legs.

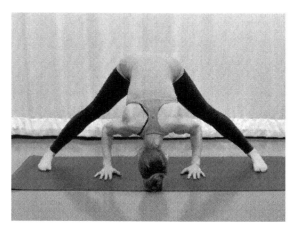

Wide-Legged Forward Fold (Prasarita Padottanasana) is similar to forward fold but is a little less intense on the hamstrings. Again, it's important to keep a flat back and lead with your chest to get the most out of this pose. To modify for tight hamstrings, place a block, chair, or some other firm object under your hands or arms so you don't fold as deeply. You can also play around with how wide you take your legs on your mat for a slightly different stretch.

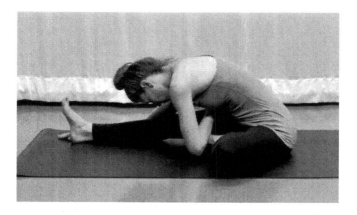

Head-to-Knee Forward Fold (Janu Sirsasana) is also a well-known hamstring stretch—you may have done this pose in gym class when you were growing up. To practice this pose, sit on your mat, extending one leg long in front of you, foot flexed. Bring the other foot to the inside of your thigh, first sitting tall, then folding forward. As in the other hamstring stretches, be sure to lead with your chest when folding in. To modify for tight hamstrings, keep a bend in the knee and don't fold over as deeply.

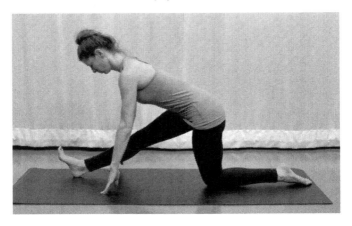

Half Monkey Pose (Ardha Hanumanasana) stretches the hamstring of the front leg. Begin in Low Lunge with your back knee on your mat, and then shift your hips back so they are stacked over your back knee. Straighten your front leg and flex your front foot. Fold forward with a flat back, bringing your chest to your front knee.

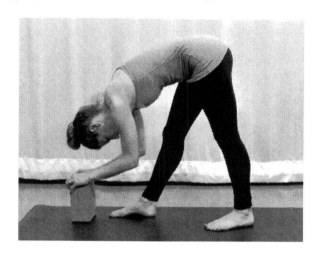

Pyramid Pose (Parsvottonasana) is a more intense hamstring stretch that you can add to your practice as you gain more flexibility. Start with your feet in Warrior I, bringing your hands to your hips. Make sure that your hips are facing squarely forward before you fold to make sure that you're getting the most out of the pose. To modify for tight hamstrings, step the back foot in closer to the front foot to shorten your stance. You can keep a bend in the front knee and you can also place something firm like a yoga block under your hands to make the pose a little easier.

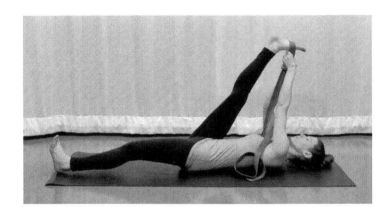

Reclined Hand-to-Big-Toe Pose (Supta Padangusthasana) can get deep into the hamstring. You can use a yoga strap if you have one, if not, use a similar object like a belt. If you're very flexible, you can grab around the big toe with your thumb, index, and middle fingers and pull your leg in with your arm. Be sure to keep your bottom foot flexed and keep that leg active and keep your back on the floor. To modify for tight hamstrings, bend the knee of the stretched leg slightly, or don't pull the leg as close to the torso.

Calf Stretches

Most runners are familiar with having tight calf muscles—they're one of the main muscles used during running, and without proper stretching they tend to get very tight. These yoga poses will help you lengthen your calf muscles, helping to release the tension in those muscles created by running.

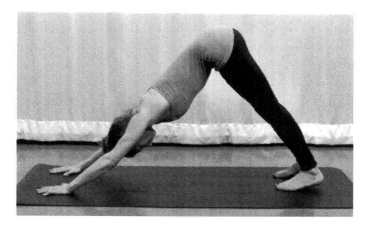

Downward Facing Dog (Adho Mukha Svanasana) is probably the best known yoga pose that stretches the calves. You can see progress over time by paying attention how close you can get your heels to your mat. Begin by bringing yourself into an inverted V, your hands shoulder-width apart and your legs hip-width apart. Melt your shoulder blades away from your ears as you pull your chest and navel closer to your thighs. As the backs of your legs begin to open, bring your heels closer to the mat. Warming up the legs by bending the knees and pedaling out your legs can help you get your heels a little closer to the mat if you're feeling stiff.

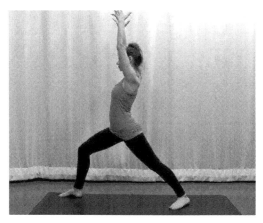

Warrior I (Virabhadrasana I) can provide a wonderful stretch through the calf of the back leg. Set up for Warrior I as described earlier, focusing on bringing your hips square, even if that means bringing your feet closer together. When your right leg is forward, think about pulling your left hip forward as you pull your right hip back to square the hips. Squaring the hips helps to intensify the stretch through the back calf muscle.

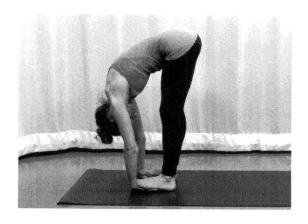

Gorilla Pose, also called **Hand Under Foot Pose (Padahastasana)** helps stretch through the calves by elevating the toes. Starting in a Standing Forward Fold, bend your knees and slide the palms of your hands under the soles of your feet. If you're very tight, try just slipping your fingertips under your toes. Your head should hang heavy as you melt forward, releasing through the backs of your legs.

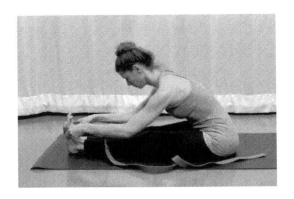

Using a strap in **Seated Forward Bend (Paschimottanasana)** is another wonderful way to stretch through the calves. Bringing the feet flexed and pulling the toes back engages the stretch in the calf muscles. In this version of the pose, it's less important to fold forward and more important to flex strongly through the feet to help deepen the calf stretch.

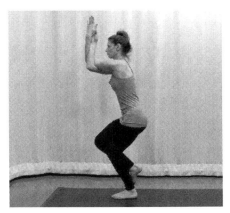

Eagle Pose (Garudasana) is less of a traditional calf stretch than the other poses, but it does stretch the calves a bit and really stretches the Achilles tendon, which runs from the calf to the heel. If the Achilles is nice and limber, it will pull less on the calf muscle, helping the calves to not feel as tight. Come into Eagle Pose on the right side by sweeping your right arm under the left as your right leg crosses over the left leg. If your shoulders are tight, wrap your hands around to opposite shoulders in a bear hug. Your right toes can stay touching the mat, you can lift your right foot, or, as you become more flexible, you can wrap your right foot around your left calf. Sink low, working to keep your elbows at shoulder height.

Poses for the Ankles and Feet

Yoga poses that act as foot stretches are fantastic for runners, especially runners training hard and/or running high mileage. Your feet and ankles literally take a pounding as you run, and the muscles, tendons, and ligaments surrounding your feet and ankles need just as much love as the ones in your legs.

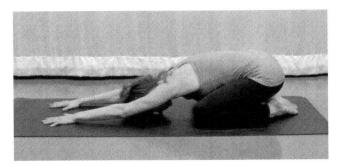

Child's Pose (Balasana) is a great warm up for deeper foot stretches. You get a nice, easy stretch through the top of your foot as it lies along the floor or a yoga mat. Try sinking your hips closer to your feet as you warm up and settle into the pose.

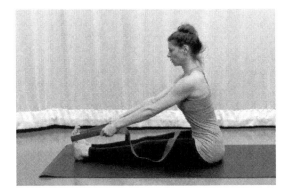

Staff Pose (Dandasana) with a strap flexes the foot and helps stretch through the heel, Achilles, and you may also feel a stretch through the calf. To come into Staff Pose, take a seat on your mat, bringing your legs long. Sit tall, lengthening through your spine. Place a yoga strap (or a belt) around the ball of your foot and gently pull on the ends of the strap. Try to keep your spine tall like you would in regular staff pose.

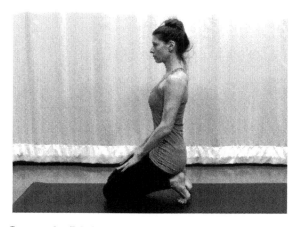

Toe Stretch (Vajrasana with curled toes) is a great foot stretch for the plantar fascia. Anyone who's had plantar fasciitis can tell you how painful it can be. Keeping your plantar fascia stretched out will help keep you from developing the nasty, painful condition. For this pose, begin in a seated position with your shins on your mat, sitting on your heels (Vajrasana). Curl your toes under as you sit back onto your heels. If this places too much pressure on your heels, place a block or a folded blanket under your seat so that some of your weight is placed on the support, off of your heels and feet. This can be a pretty intense foot stretch, so only hold the pose as long as is comfortable. You can come into the pose a few times in a row, resting your feet and ankles in between.

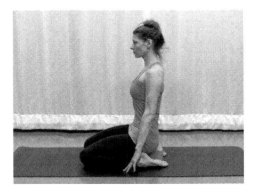

Hero Pose (Virasana) is an intense foot stretch for the top of the feet. This pose can be hard on the knees, so if you have bad knees you'll want to modify or possibly avoid doing this pose.

Begin by kneeling with the tops of your feet on your mat, then bring your feet slightly wider than your hips. Sit down, bringing your hips between your feet; your heels will be on either side of your hips. You can modify the pose by sitting on a yoga block or a folded blanket. Again, hold this intense stretch for as long as comfortable, doing multiple rounds of the pose when your feet need some extra stretching.

CHAPTER 6
Yoga Poses for the Core

Having good core strength is so important to help maintain proper running form. A strong core will help you avoid leaning too far forward or back as you run, and will help you support your entire body as you run. So, it makes sense that having good core strength as a runner is incredibly important. These yoga poses will help you maintain and increase core strength, helping you keep proper running form even as you get tired.

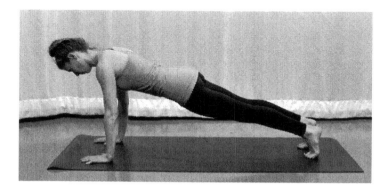

Many people think of **Plank Pose (Kumbhakasana)** when they think of core strengthening yoga poses. It's a wonderful pose for the core because it helps to make the muscles all the way around the core stronger. In Plank Pose, be sure to stack your hands directly beneath your shoulders and keep your abs pulled in, which will help you keep your hips in line with your shoulders and heels. If you're not strong enough to hold a full plank, you can start with keeping your knees on the ground and work up from there.

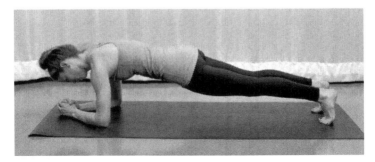

Dolphin Plank (Makara Adho Mukha Svanasana) is a wonderful plank variation if you have bad wrists. Come to your hands and knees, clasp your hands together in front of you, keeping your elbows at shoulder width, stacking your elbows under your shoulders. Curl your toes under, lifting you knees off the ground. Engage your core as you bring your hips in line with your shoulders like you did in Plank Pose.

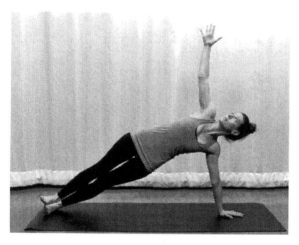

Side Plank (Vasisthasana) also helps work the entire core, but puts a greater emphasis on the obliques. Begin in Plank Pose, rotating your weight to one hand, which stacks under your shoulder. Come to the knife edge of your bottom foot, stacking the top foot directly over the bottom foot if you can. Stack your shoulders and hips over one another, then pull your core in, lifting your hips high to engage your obliques.

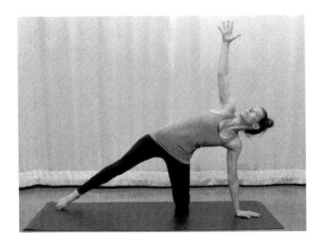

Until you work up to full Side Plank, you can keep your bottom knee on the floor. If you have bad wrists, either keep your knee on the floor, or if you have both legs lifted, you can come to the forearm of your supporting arm. Once you've built enough strength, you can try lifting your top leg to intensify the pose.

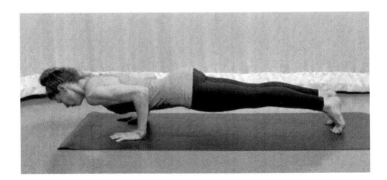

Low Plank (Chaturanga Dandasana) is great at strengthening the core and the shoulders. From Plank Pose, shift your body forward as your hands stay planted, then lower down so your elbows are in line with your shoulders. Be sure to keep your elbows snugly in to your sides, with your upper arms grazing your ribcage. Like in Plank Pose, you can practice this pose on your knees until you build up the strength for full Low Plank.

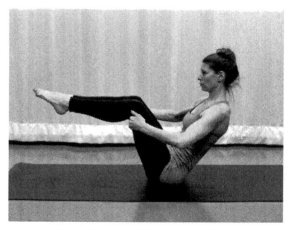

Boat pose (Paripurna Navasana) is really wonderful for working the entire core. To practice Boat Pose, start in a seated position. Place your hands behind your thighs and rock back, balancing on your seat. Engage your core as you lean back, making a V with your upper body and thighs. Start with your toes on the ground, then try bending your knees and bringing them to a tabletop position. You can bring your arms straight in front of you or up by your ears. When you build enough strength, you can come into full Boat Pose by extending your legs straight.

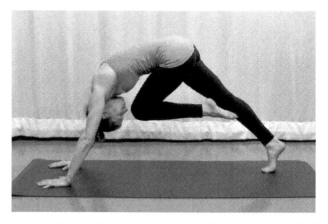

Knee to Nose is a Downward Facing Dog (Adho Mukha Svanasana) modification that is great for strengthening the core. Start in Downward Facing Dog, then bring your feet to meet, lined up with the middle of your hips. Inhale your heel high, then pull your knee in toward your nose as you gaze back, pulling your abs in and engaging your core. You can play around with taking the knee to either elbow to work different parts of your abs.

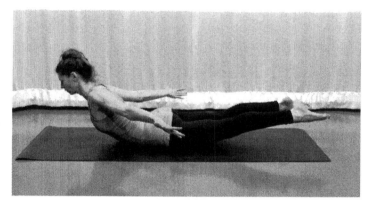

Locust Pose (Salabhasana) is fantastic for strengthening your lower back. If you do a lot of abdominal exercises, it's also important to work the lower back so that the muscles on the front and back sides of your body don't become imbalanced. Begin by lying on your stomach, with your legs long below you and your arms at your sides. Lift your chest and legs off your mat, engaging the muscles in your back. Lift the upper and lower body higher to intensify, or stay lower if you need to modify.

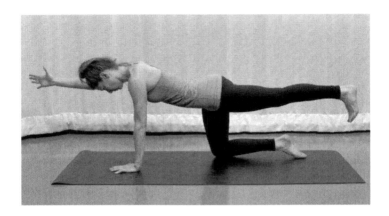

Balancing Table Pose is another great way to engage your core and strengthen your lower back. Begin in a tabletop position with your hands stacked below your shoulders and your knees stacked below your hips. Inhale your right heel to hip height, flexing through your foot. To intensify, bring your left arm up by your ear. Hold for a few breaths, then carefully lower your hand and leg back to tabletop before switching to the other side.

Core and Spinal Flexibility

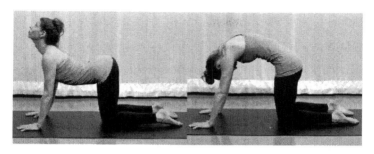

Flowing between **Cat (Marjaryasana)** and **Cow (Bitilasana) Poses** is a wonderful way to warm up the spine and increase spinal flexibility. Begin in a tabletop position, then on an inhale, let your navel fall toward your mat as your seat and gaze go toward the ceiling for **Cow Pose**. On your exhale, pull your lower back up toward the ceiling as you gaze back toward your thighs, pulling your hips under for **Cat Pose**. You can flow through Cat and Cow Poses with your breath, coming to Cow Pose on your inhales and Cat Pose on your exhales.

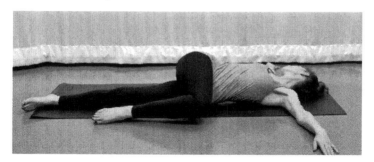

Supine Twist (Supta Matsyendrasana) helps to stretch your lower spine. Begin by lying on your back, then bring your right knee to your right armpit. Keeping both shoulders pressed firmly into the mat, let your right knee fall to the left. You can bring a block or blanket under your right knee for extra support. Your gaze can stay up to the ceiling, or fall to the right toward your right hand. Be sure to hold the pose on the left side for an equal length of time.

CHAPTER 7
Heart Openers

Good running form involves not only the lower body and core, but also the upper body and shoulders. If your shoulders are rounded and hunched over, you'll have a greater tendency to lean forward, creating an inefficient gait. Opening your chest and shoulders with these heart opening yoga poses will allow you to run with better posture, helping you maintain good form.

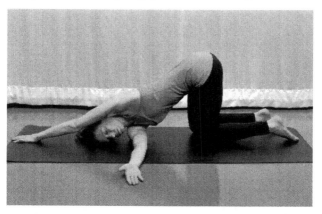

Thread the Needle Pose (Parsva Balasana) helps to open the backs of the shoulders.

Starting from a tabletop position, walk your left hand forward on the mat, extending it long while still keeping your hips stacked over your knees. Reach your right arm through the hole beneath your left arm, allowing the back of your shoulder to rest on the mat. Repeat on the other side.

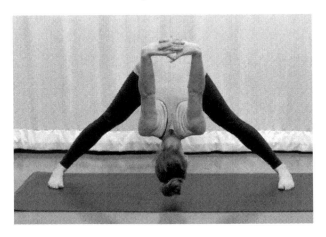

The bind in **Wide Legged Forward Fold with Bind (Prasarita Padottanasana C)** helps to pull the shoulders back and open the chest muscles. Start with your legs wide on the mat, like setting up for a standard Wide Legged Forward Fold. Clasp your hands behind your back, using a towel or a strap between your hands if you have tight shoulders. Straighten your arms, then fold forward with a flat back, letting your hands fall toward your mat. Listen to your body—if the bind starts to feel like it's too much on your shoulders, release it.

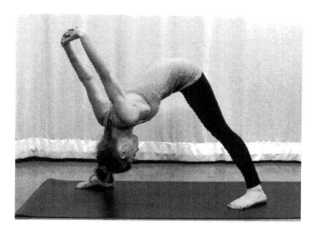

Humble Warrior (Baddha Virabhadrasana) also incorporates a bind that helps to open the shoulders and heart. Starting in Warrior I, clasp your hands behind you. As with the previous pose, you can use a strap or a towel to help you access the bind if your shoulders are tight. Hinge forward from the waist with a flat back, bringing your shoulders inside your front knee. Melt down, letting your head hang heavy, releasing your neck.

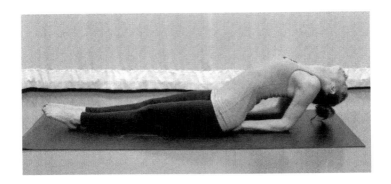

Fish Pose (Matsyasana) helps open the heart and the throat. To come into Fish Pose, begin by sitting on your mat with your legs long in front of you. Slide your hands under your tailbone, bringing your index fingers and thumbs together in a diamond shape. Prop yourself up on your elbows, then gently let your head fall back. If you're very flexible the crown of your head may touch the yoga mat. You may find that it's more comfortable to breathe through your mouth for this pose than through your nose.

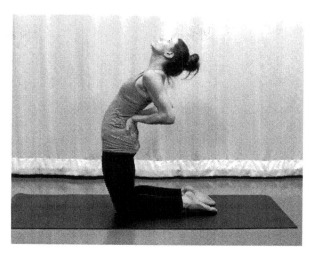

Camel Pose (Ustrasana) is a great heart opener as well as a good stretch for the front side of your hips. Begin in a kneeling position with your knees stacked under your hips. Bring your hands on your lower back, placing them where your back pockets would be. Use your hands to support your lower back as you gently lean back, being careful to not force your neck back. Continue to press your hips forward, keeping them stacked over your knees.

CHAPTER 8
Balancing Poses

Balancing yoga poses are really great for strengthening stabilizer muscles, especially in the standing leg. They'll help strengthen your foot and your ankle, which will reduce your risk of getting sprains when you misstep. Strengthening your arch can help reduce your risk of getting the dreaded plantar fasciitis. And, balancing will strengthen the rest of your leg, your hips, and your core. Balancing will also help you improve your mental focus, since a lot of focus is required to hold balancing poses for a longer period of time. One side is often more difficult to balance on, so try not to focus on one side being "better" than the other. Instead, try to focus on just experiencing the pose for what it is.

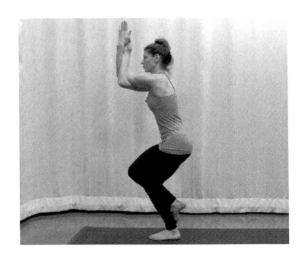

Eagle Pose (Garudasana) not only strengthens the ankle and foot, but it's also a good stretch for the Achilles and ankle of the standing leg. If you're just starting to work on balancing poses, keep the toes of the top leg on the ground next to the outside of your standing leg as a kickstand. As you get better at this pose, start to lift the toes of the top leg off the ground and gradually work on wrapping the foot around your standing ankle. If you have tight shoulders, skip the wrapped arm variation and just give yourself a bear hug.

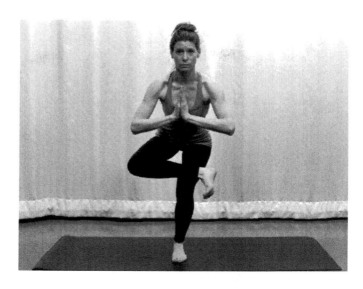

Standing Pigeon Pose, also called **Figure Four Pose (Eka Pada Utkatasana)** is a wonderful pose for runners because you stretch through the hip and glute of the non-standing leg, places where runners tend to get really tight. You're stretching many of the same muscles you stretch in regular pigeon pose with the added benefit of strengthening your ankle and foot. Flex strongly through the foot of the top leg and sink lower to intensify the stretch. Think about pulling the top knee down and back, too, if you want to deepen the stretch a little more.

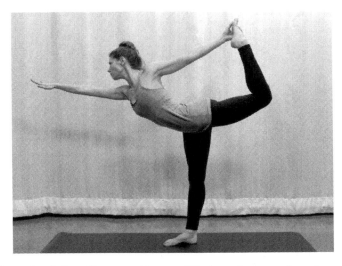

Lord of the Dance Pose (Natarajasana) not only helps you strengthen the foot and ankle of your standing leg, but it also helps to open the hip flexor of the back leg. Come into Lord of the Dance Pose by grounding down through your left foot, which creates a solid base in the left foot, then shifting your weight into your left leg. Your left arm comes straight up by your ear. Bend your right knee and bring your right heel close to your glutes, then grab the inside of your right foot with your right hand. Kick your right foot into your right hand, having the option to stand tall or to lean forward. Switch sides before finishing.

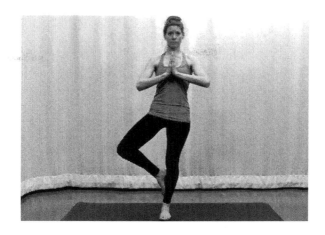

Tree Pose (Vrksasana) is a great balancing pose for runners because it can also help to open the hips. Begin by standing at the top of your mat, shifting your weight into your left foot. Bring your right foot up to your left leg, either keeping your right heel at your left ankle and your toes on the mat, bringing your right foot to your left calf, or bringing your right foot up to the left thigh. Try to avoid bringing your foot to your knee, which can put extra stress on the knee joint. Press your standing leg into your foot just as much as you press your foot into your leg to create a solid base. Play around with angling your heel slightly forward and your toes slightly back to experience a greater opening in the hips. You have many options for your arms, including keeping them heart center, raising them up overhead, or even keeping them by your sides, fingertips wide. After holding on the left for a few breaths, switch sides.

CHAPTER 9
Restorative Yoga Poses for Runners

One way yoga can really help runners is by aiding recovery. Restorative yoga poses help release the tension that builds in muscle and connective tissue, helping you maintain a good range of motion. These poses can also help promote proper blood flow, which aids the removal of waste products from tissues and brings in oxygen and nutrients. This chapter features my favorite restorative yoga for runners poses that I use to recover from my running. Hold each of these poses for two to three minutes, or as long as it's comfortable.

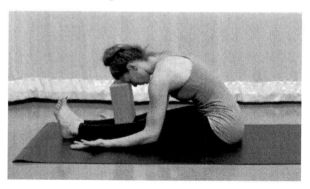

A **Supported Seated Forward Fold (Paschimottanasana)** is wonderful for opening up the hamstrings, making it a perfect yoga for runners pose. The key to making this a restorative pose is to stack blocks, pillows, blankets, or other supportive items under your chest and/or head so that you can relax your upper body. If you find that you're putting weight on your arms, flip your hands over so that the palms face up—this can help you relax a little deeper. Be very careful that you're gently stretching through the belly of the hamstrings (the thick, meaty part of the muscle) and that it feels like a gentle stretch, not like you're straining.

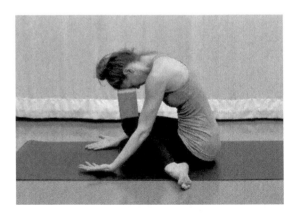

Cow Face Forward Fold (Gomukhasana
variation) is great for opening and stretching the
outer thigh and leg, especially the piriformis,
which tends to be a problem area for a lot of
runners. You stack your knees together, bringing
your feet out to the side. If you bring your feet
closer to your hips, you'll deepen the stretch, but
remember, you should be relaxing into these
poses, so there's no need to push. Support your
head and/or chest with blocks, blankets, etc. as
needed.

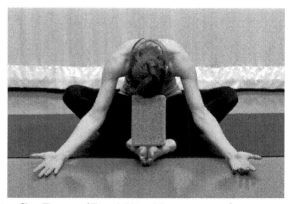

Butterfly Pose (Baddha Konasana)
counteracts cow face pose by opening up the
inner thigh. You press the soles of your feet
together and let your knees go out wide. Your

feet can be as close to or far away from your hips as they need to be to make the pose comfortable. Again, use props to support your torso so that you can relax into the pose.

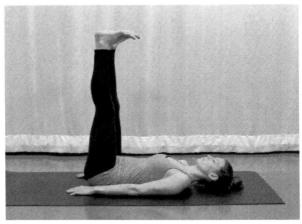

Legs up the Wall (Viparita Karani) is a perennial favorite of runners because it helps drain waste products from running and muscle breakdown from the legs and helps bring fresh blood in when you bring your legs down after the pose. Lying on your side, you should try to get your seat as close as you can to the wall. Then, flip onto your back, letting your legs rest against the wall. Hold the pose for about five minutes, less if the pose is uncomfortable.

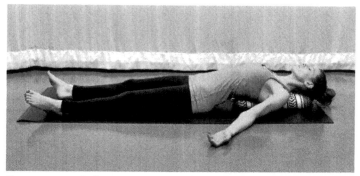

Supported Corpse Pose (Savasana) is a wonderful heart opener. You see it all the time on the running path: may runners have a tendency to run with hunched shoulders. This pose helps counteract the hunching by opening up the muscles on the front side of your shoulder, including the pectorals. By placing a bolster, folded blanket, or even a yoga mat under your spine between your shoulders, it allows your heart and shoulders to open. Allow the tension to melt out of your muscles as you relax into the mat. This pose is a wonderful final resting pose after a yoga practice, allowing you to recenter yourself mentally and physically.